Grandma's Natural Remedies and Ancient Herbal Recipes -Vol 4

Herbs, Spices, And Tips To Keep Healthy

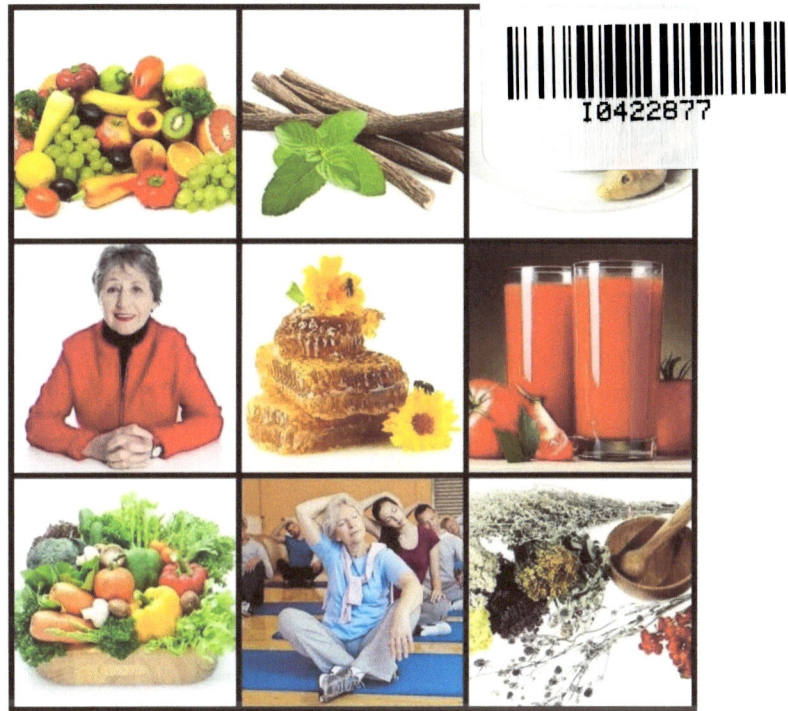

Dueep Jyot Singh
Natural Remedy Series
Mendon Cottage Books

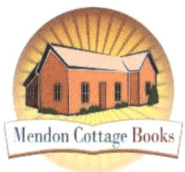

JD-Biz Publishing

Disclaimer

The information is this book is provided for informational purposes only. It is not intended to be used and medical advice or a substitute for proper medical treatment by a qualified health care provider. The information is believed to be accurate as presented based on research by the author.

The contents have not been evaluated by the U.S. Food and Drug Administration or any other Government or Health Organization and the contents in this book are not to be used to treat cure or prevent disease.

The author or publisher is not responsible for the use or safety of any diet, procedure, or treatment mentioned in this book. The author or publisher is not responsible for errors or omissions that may exist.

Warning

The Book is for informational purposes only and before taking on any diet, treatment, or medical procedure, it is recommended to consult with your primary health care provider.

Our books are available at

1. Amazon.com

2. Barnes and Noble

3. Itunes

4. Kobo

5. Smashwords

6. Google Play Books

Table of Contents

Introduction

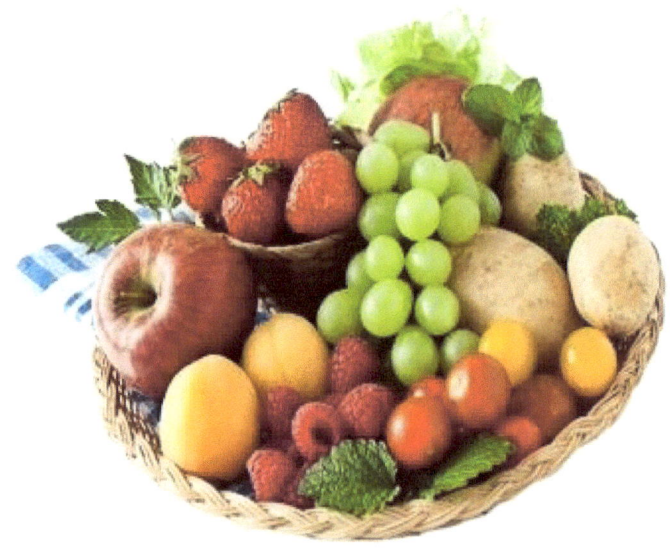

In this fourth volume of grandma's ancient natural remedies and herbal recipes, you are going to get a collection of recipes, in which grandmother used fruit, vegetables, herbs and spices to cure her family and also the neighbors around her.

These remedies were given to her down the ages from our grandmother, and so on. Many of these remedies have been lost in the mists of time, but there were still some people in ancient times who wrote these remedies down in books.

In 800 BC, Homer praised the knowledge of ancient Egyptians, who were extremely skilled in noninvasive surgery, and treatment of ailments. Ancient well-known Greek and Roman medicine men like Galen and Hippocratus gained plenty of their knowledge studying in the University of Amenhotep and the great and glorious physician Lucanus – known in Biblical history as Saint Luke – studied under Greek and Egyptian physicians.

There were plenty of physicians who believe in spells, and considered that disease was caused by evil demons. Tibetan and other Eastern medicine still uses incantations to get rid of demons which have possessed a human or an animal body, thus causing it to get sick.

In Indian and Chinese medicine, the ancient doctors had a good knowledge of the human anatomy. More than 4000 years ago, doctors in India were practicing plastic surgery, by making up noses from flaps of skin taken from other parts of the body. In the same manner, Chinese doctors knew all about blood circulation and acupuncture.

In fact, Chinese medicine can be considered to be one of the most ancient, scientific and knowledgeable science ever known to mankind in today's world. It was well documented, as was Egyptian medicine, of which many ancient priceless papyrii have been found.

Many of these ancient doctors knew about cause and effect, even though the belief of disease causing demons possessing a body still lingers on in many parts of the East. People are also under the impression that diseases are under the control and power of gods and goddesses who have to be placated so that they do not send an epidemic in the coming rainy season.

Egypt, China, Greece, Mesopotamia, and India were fertile lands. That is why there was absolutely no reason why the people living here could not have plenty of healthy food to eat. Grains, fruit, vegetables, cereals, spices, nuts, and other natural health giving food were in abundance. This is why the ancients lived so long. Because of this healthy natural diet, and most of the people living outdoors, ailments and illnesses were few.

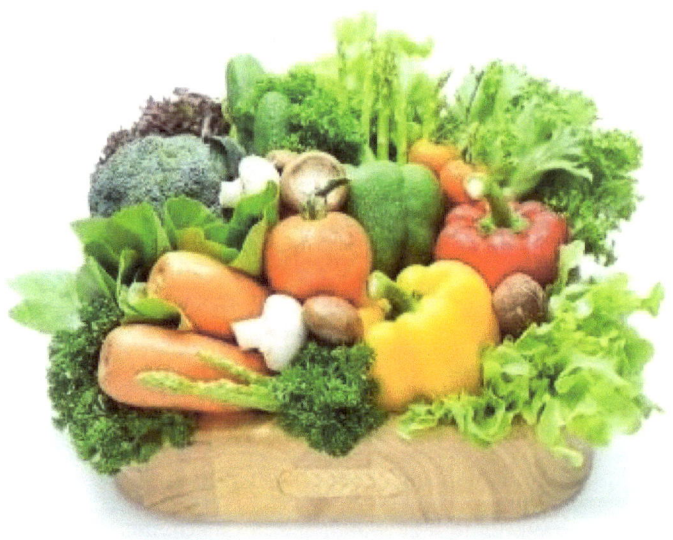

That is why people of the 21st century are coming back to nature and looking for natural remedies based on fruit and vegetables, which are going to cure them of diseases and ailments. Chemical-based drugs may heal you very well on a short-term basis, but they are going to have an everlasting long-term effect on your body. That is because they are made up of chemicals, which do not suit the biophysiological functioning system of your body.

On the other hand, fruits and vegetables as well as herbs are going to heal your body naturally, while making sure that you do not suffer from any sort of side effects. This is the reason why grandma 's collected herbal lore and knowledge is all about the wonderful medical and beauty enhancing benefits of different herbs, spices, fruit, vegetables and flowers.

What is The Importance Of Fruit, Vegetables, Herbs And Spices?

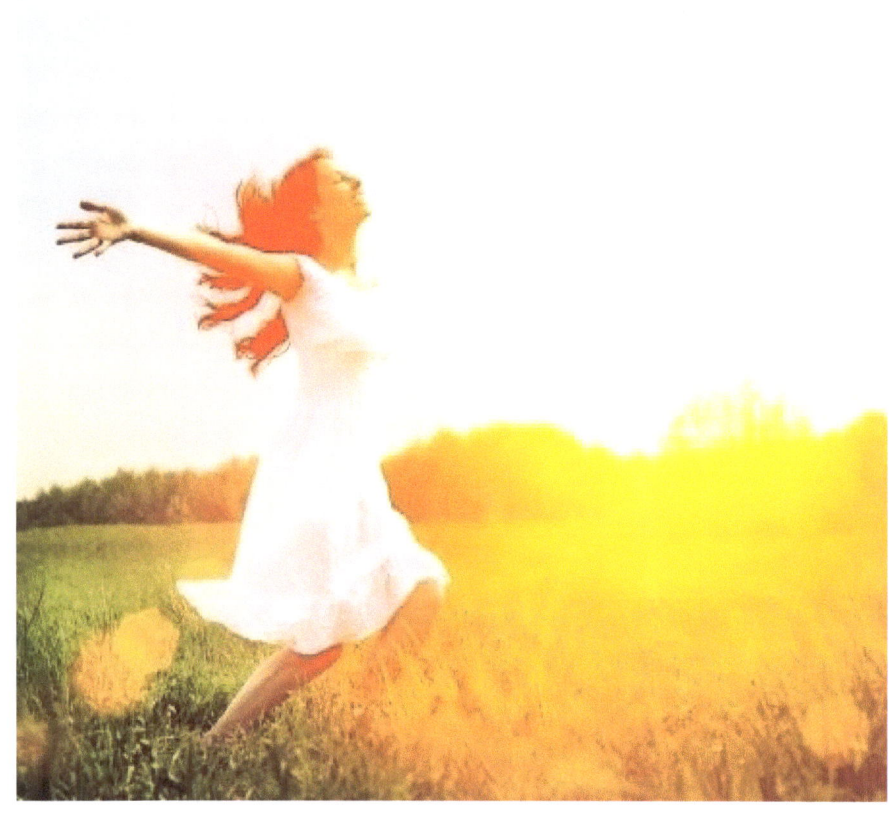

Remember – good health is your birthright!

Natural means everything readily available in nature – including fruit, vegetables, minerals, water, fresh air and even sunlight.

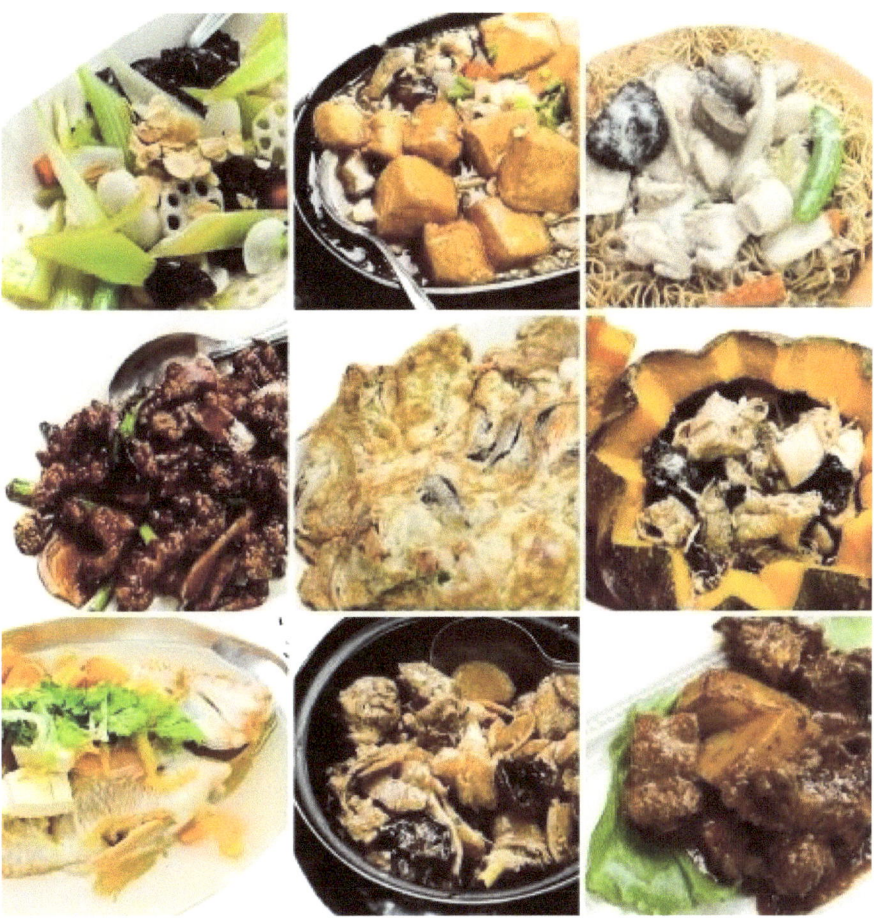

These are comparatively modern preparations, but the basic ingredients – herbs, vegetables, meat, spices and cereals have been in use for millenniums all over the world.

In ancient times, wise men advocated the addition of fresh fruit and vegetables to our diet, because even though man is naturally omnivorous, – with a natural innate predilection towards meat, fish and other high-protein foods – fruit and vegetables were considered to be easier to digest, and much healthier. In fact if you look at the diet of the ancients of long ago, their food was mostly cereal-based with lots of dairy products including Goat's milk, camels' milk and the milk from cows, yaks, buffaloes and other bovines. These were made into butter, yogurt and cheese.

Cereals were made into breads, or fermented into beer. Spices were used to heal diseases, as well as to season foods. Flowers were used for ornamentation and decoration purposes, as well as the medium for extracting aromatic oils used for medical and beauty purposes.

Did you know that the ancients daily diet consisted of 20% fruit and vegetables? We have forgotten this wise practice today, because first of all, we would rather eat meat than eat fruit and vegetables. Why is this so? Here is the psychological reason. Since childhood, we have been indoctrinated with our elders telling us to eat our veggies because it is good for us. This naturally makes us subconsciously not want to eat veggies. On the other hand, if they had told us, not to eat some particular fruit or veggie, because it was not good for us, we would immediately make that particular natural product a major part of our daily diet. That is because mankind is naturally perverse in nature, and stubborn enough not to follow a thing, because somebody said so.

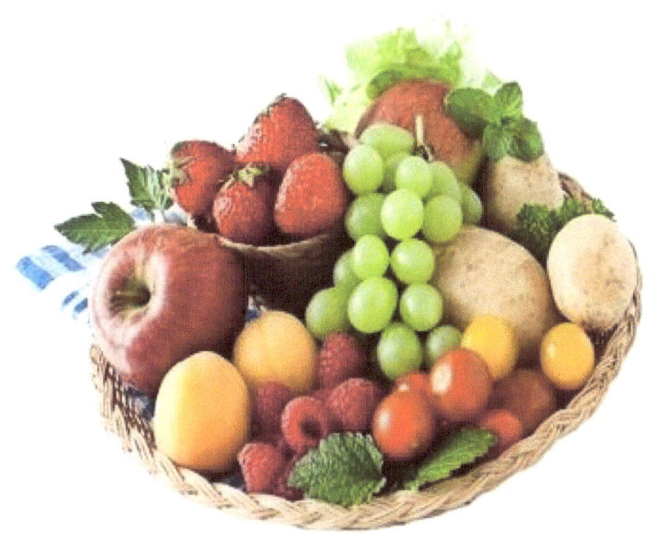

More fruit in your diet is good for you

So remember that fruit and vegetables are not "boring grasses and fodder fit only for cattle" – a statement made by one of my acquaintances as he polished off a juicy steak smothered in potatoes and onions – instead, they are an interesting and healthy, tasty supplement to our diet, which could otherwise easily become monotonous and unhealthy.

It is a sad fact that nearly all the POWs in concentration camps, when rescued were found to be advanced cases of malnutrition. That is because they did not have anything green, yellow or red to eat. No question of the ever being fed seeds and nuts unless they found some growing in their camps. No lemons meant that they would suffer from beriberi. No greens meant no vitamins. Not many cereals meant no other essential nutrients.

So remember that grandmother used raw vegetables in salads. Boiled and grilled vegetables were normally given to invalids or finicky eaters. Along with that fruit and vegetables were used to develop amazing traditional cuisines, which came down through generations in a large variety of boiled, grilled, baked, braised, fried, minced and broiled dishes where fruit and vegetables played a major part.

In ancient times, grandma either went into her garden or went to the nearest vegetable market in order to pick the freshest choicest items at the best rate. Nowadays, we go to the nearest store and pick up the most easily grabbed preserved food package with a shelf life which says it can be kept in our fridge for 6 months.

Also, we believe in bulk buying. That is because we think we are getting bargains of 2% off, by buying 5 pounds of fruit, which may have just come out of cold storage and may not be able to withstand the harsh rigors of more storage in the fresh air, because their natural shelf life is over.

Grandma definitely did not cook for an army. She knew exactly how much food she needed to prepare to feed her hungry brood. Nowadays, people make the mistake of overestimating the amount of food required by their families and there goes the left over food right into the refrigerator. You may find some of this food growing mold after a couple of weeks, if it has been placed in a remote corner in your refrigerator. Grandma was much more sensible. If there were any leftovers left, she would feed them to the livestock at the end of the meal or at the end of the day. The next day started with a brand-new menu with fresh ingredients.

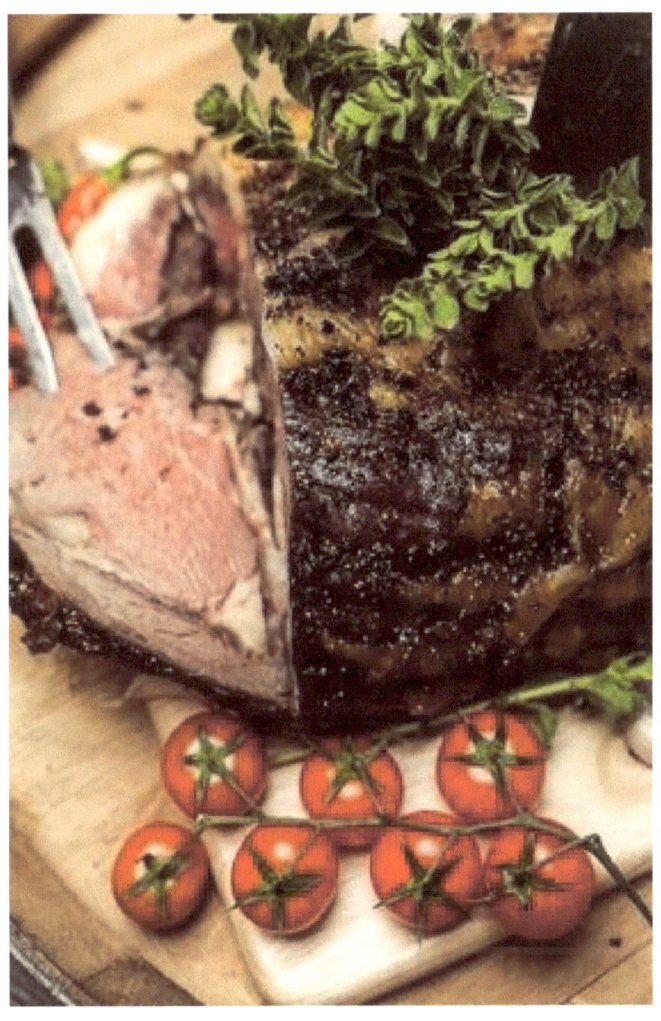

Grandma used plenty of fresh ingredients to cook delicious meals for her family.

If you want to store food, remember that apples and lettuces are going to go bad if there are any bad brown spots on their surfaces. Remember the say about bad apples and remove the spots before storing. The rest of the apples and the lettuces are going to keep much longer, because the rotten apples and lettuces have been thrown out into the livestock troughs.

Spices and Herbs in Your Daily Diet

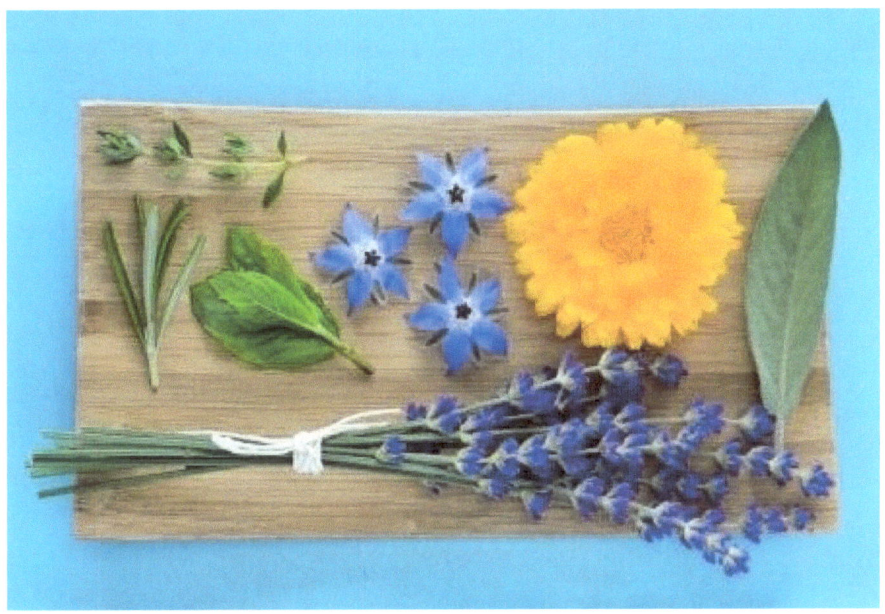

Grandma was very careful about the quantity of spices that she used in her cuisine. The idea of masala mixtures – garam masala, curry masala-preserved in oil is a comparatively new idea which came in existence in the late 18th century, when British traders were given the idea to preserve these ground spices in oil and take them home to Blighty. That is why the curry masala or Mussaman masala you get in convenience stores near you, is dripping in oil, with the spices mixed in it willy-nilly. You do not even know about the proportions of the spices used. So it is much better to collect your own spices, and grind them whenever required. Remember that ground spices made up into a masala is going to lose its aroma and power after a little while.

If you are living in the East, and are used to cooking Eastern dishes, it is possible that you are still roasting spices in a small pan, prior to grinding them. This supposedly fixed the flavor. After that, you would sprinkle the garam masala – not more than one – 2 teaspoons – over the prepared masala while preparing a dish [Original cooking masala base, which would be made up of onion, garlic, tomatoes, rocksalt and turmeric].

This last mixing of garam masala was done to add the extra spice to the cooking masala mixture.

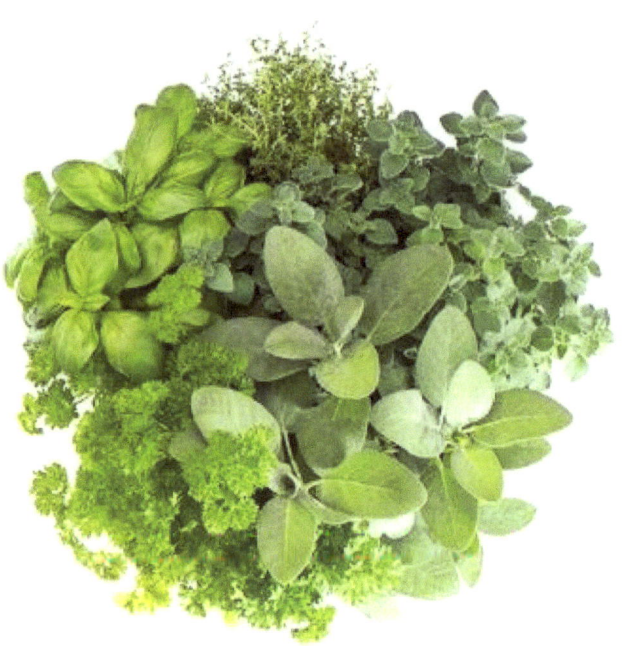

Many people trying out an Eastern dish for the first time are under the impression that garam masala is fried, along with the onions, garlic, and other spices. Not so. It is added after the onions etc. are golden Brown and fried properly. Consider garam masala to be a healthy digestive additive added to the dish, while cooking.

In the West, you of course cannot do without Parsley, Cilantro, Rosemary, Thyme, Sage, Dill and other delicious and healthy herbs added to your cuisine. You would them automatically in your dishes, without even considering their power. That is because you have seen people cooking these dishes in front of you, who automatically did that same action. This is subconscious. This is also how knowledge was passed on from generation to generation and is still being passed on to future generations.

Grandma – Cook and Medicine Woman

Grandmother was half a medicine woman herself. She knew that some spices were "hot"and some spices were "cold". These are just some of the spices and herbs which are used to heal and in cuisine.

Asafoetida, Aniseed, Fennel, Fenugreek, Bishops Weed – also known as lovage – Lemongrass, Lime, Ginger, Mint, Nutmeg, Mustard Seeds, Paprika, Poppy Seeds, Pimento, Dill seeds, Turmeric, Rosemary, Thyme, Sesame, Saffron, Mustard, Nutmeg, Cinnamon, Cloves, Coriander, Cumin Seeds, Fennel, Caraway, Cardamom, Chilies, Coriander Seeds... Whew.

And we have only just begun. Each of them had their own medical and curative properties. Each of them were used in some medical preparation or the other. Some plants, herbs and spices alas have been forgotten by mankind, because they have become extinct or all knowledge of them has disappeared from the face of the earth. But we are lucky that we can manage to make do with what we have right now. If I lived in medieval times, I would have understood what the dishes or spices meant. But alas, I can just read and marvel. Behold, the times of William the Conqueror...

"...*when Raoul admitted that my lord Robert had been troubled lately by coughs she was able at once to tell him of a remedy which the Duchess Matilda (being a foreigner) might not know.*

'You must pluck a sprig of mistletoe grown over a thornbush,' she said earnestly. 'This being soaked in the milk of a mare and given to my lord Robert to drink it, he will cough no more.'

Raoul made a polite response. Gisela began to eat of a Lombardy leach, flourished and served with a sober-sauce, but she did not eat much of it because her quick eye had observed all manner of delicate dishes on the board, and she meant to taste of as many as she was able. She glanced round her, and wondered aloud whether the Lady Adeline would instruct her in the way to make appulmoy, and whether it were well to put a dash of cubebs in a blank desire. One of the scullions had just brought in a dish of curlews. Gisela finished up what was left on her platter in a hurry. The curlews were served with chaldron, and Gisela was occupied for some time in trying to make up her mind whether this was flavoured with canelle, or powder-douce. Raoul could not help her, but she presently decided that there must be a dash of each in it, and perhaps a few grains of Paradise, as well. She became aware of Raoul's silence suddenly, and saw him staring down at the dregs of his hippocras...[1]"

Later on, the hero Raoul would stretch out his hand towards a dish of petypanel, and begin to nibble a piece of it reflectively.

Now all of these dishes, and herbs are exotic, but who knows how to cook them or knows about these spices? Not I, for sure. But grandma knew them and used them, and was curious enough to know what went into which he dish, to give it to that distinct aroma and flavor.

Grandma not only used herbs and spices as medicines to cure ailments, but she also used these herbs and spices in cuisine.

Garam Masala Recipe

If you want to make the original garam masala recipe, which has come down down the ages, you need to collect 1 teaspoon each of fennel seeds, cloves, cardamom, lovage – also known As Bishops Weed, and ground

---

[1] Georgette Heyer-<u>The Conqueror</u>.

nutmeg. Now these spices together consisted of hot and cold. Some of them were winter spices, to be eaten in winter to produce heat in the body. Others were summer spices to be eaten in summer, to cool the body. Now cinnamon and cloves are considered to be "hot. "That is why they are made into tea masala and drunk in the winter.

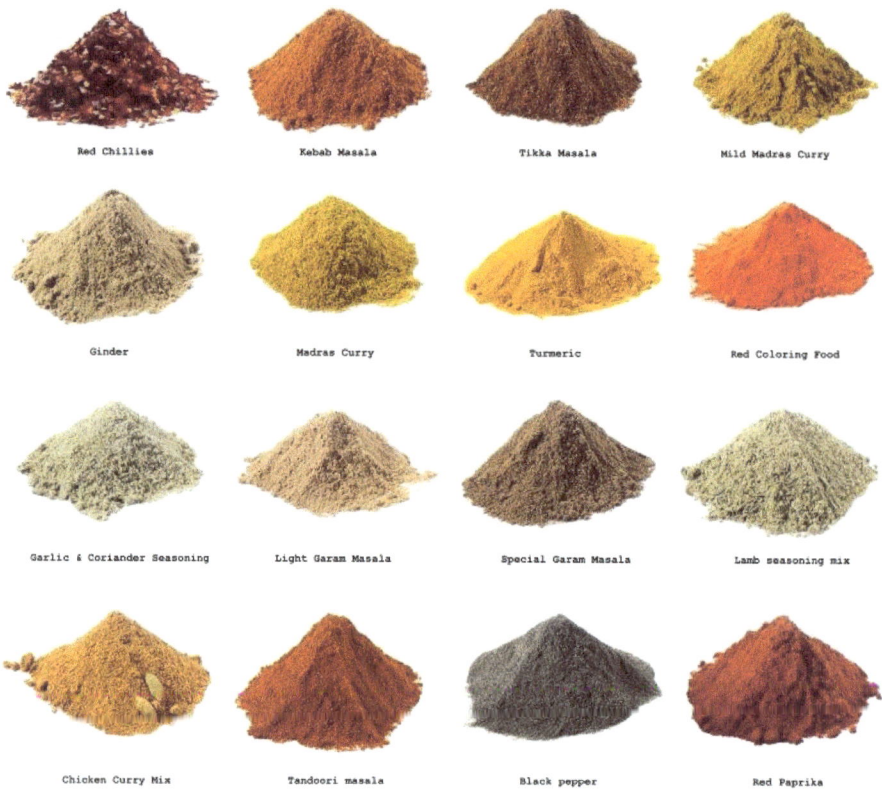

Imagine! All these masalas are just different combinations of spices in different proportions. Seems like a masala for every dish and for every use.

The spices were fried separately and put in a pan. After that, you fried 3 tablespoons full of coriander seeds, and 1 ½ tablespoonfuls of cumin seeds. You ground all of these together in a grinder or in a mortar – mortar grinding is considered to be a part of Eastern cuisine, even today – along with 3 2 inch pieces of cinnamon, powdered.

Strain and filter the powder and place in airtight glass jar. This is going to keep for three months, but it is not at all as powerful and potent as the freshly ground masala, made by your own hand. No wonder one of my chef friends nearly brained me with a heavy cooking ladle, when I asked him in all innocence whether he used garam masala and Mussaman masala while cooking oriental dishes.

Use just a teaspoon of this garam masala in your cuisine to give it the authentic Oriental Taste.

Massaman Masala

Grandmothers in Korea were so well versed in herbal and spice lore, that the royal family used a medicine woman to cook food for them. Every day she used to make up a new menu, to keep the whole royal family healthy, keeping in view the biophysiological and chemical makeup of each individual.

Grandmas in Thailand Thailand also knew about the healing and curative properties of spices. That is why they made sure that the Curryies they made had just that perfect blend of sweet, sour, hot and spicy taste. The ingredients used to make the Massaman curry paste was made up of four small, chopped and seeded red chilies, 2 teaspoons each of fresh lemongrass, sugar and peanut oil, 3 chopped green shallots and four cloves of crushed garlic. To this mixture was added half a teaspoon each of turmeric, cinnamon, cumin, cloves and cardamom. A paste was made by blending all these ingredients with water.

You may notice that some spices are more in quantity, while others are less. This is what brings about the balance of the right healing and curative power of these spices, according to ancient medicine. That is the reason why some spices were used in excess, like coriander, while others were used in smaller quantities like cloves, cardamom, cinnamon, and lovage.

So do not go overboard when you are making your own spice mixtures. Stick to authentic traditional recipes. You may find yourself suffering from prickly heat in the summer, if you used garam masala made up of large quantities of cinnamon, cloves and cardamom. That is why grandmothers in the East never fed their families with spicy foods in the summer.

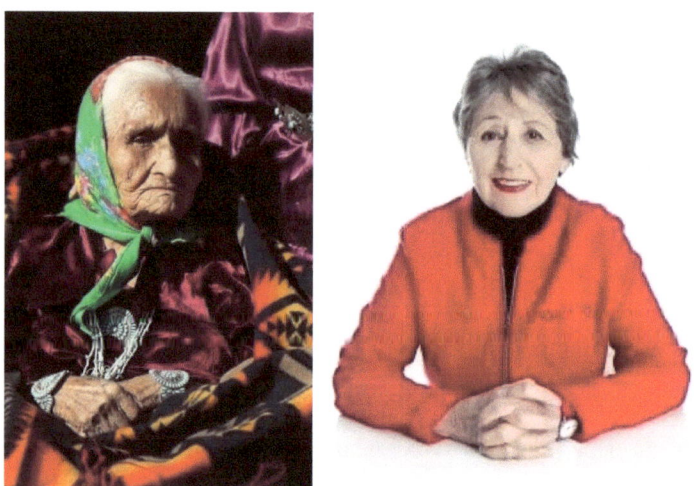

It does not matter whether grandmas are traditional or modern – it is their knowledge and experience that counts in today's world.

Grandma's Herbal Tips

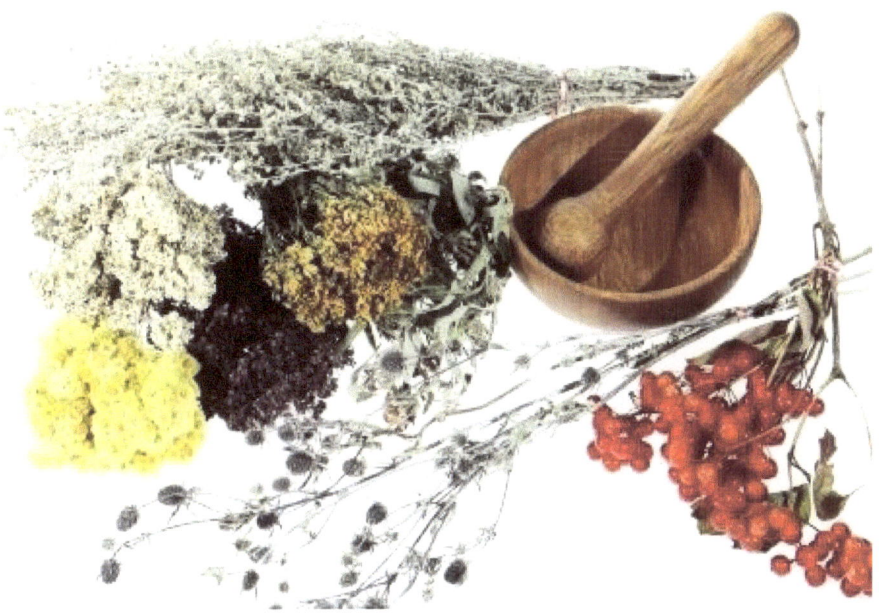

Here are some of grandma's herbal tips which are easy to follow, especially when you are far away from a doctor. She used them to keep her family healthy. Some of them may not have any scientific basis, but they have been in use for centuries. That is why anybody willing to do research on them can look at the possible reasons for such success.

Controlling High Blood Pressure

I am so glad that I was not born in medieval times. The moment I lost my temper, or got a bit het up, I would immediately be cupped and bled. That was exactly how backward European medical science was up to the 19th century. In Regency times, the moment any aristocrat, but emotionally disturbed, he would call for his barber, who would immediately open up a vein. A pint or so of blood would thus be removed, and by that time, the patient would be so weak, that he would consider that he had been cured.

In fact, it is a sad historical fact that Princess Charlotte, the future ruler of England, and the only daughter of Prinny – King George the fourth of England – died supposedly at childbirth, but more due to the extreme ignorance and stupidity of her doctor. He cupped her regularly during her pregnancy, because he considered her to be fat and he had an idea that this was the only way in which she could bear a healthy child. No wonder she died.

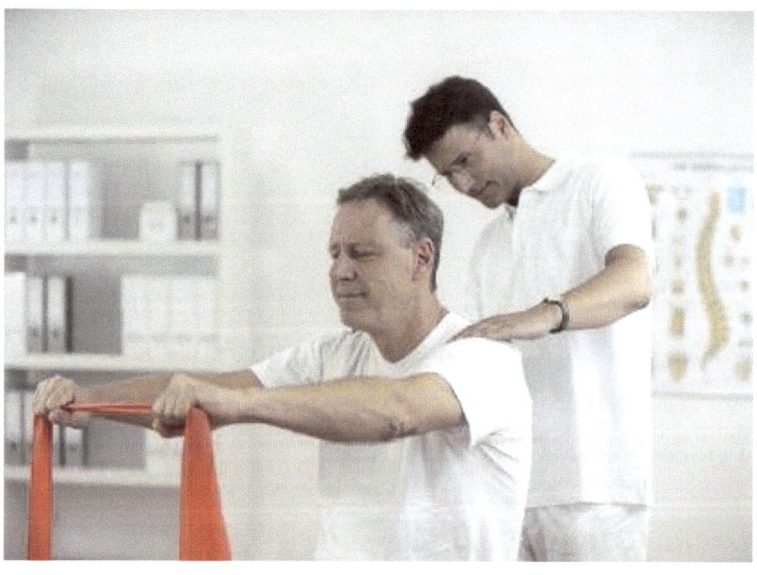

HBP is known as the silent killer. So remember to get a regular checkup.

Anyway, it is not surprising that such ignorant people thought that high blood pressure could be reduced by cupping. But they definitely did not change their lifestyle, which included eating, drinking and making merry, every evening, without fail. Meals at that time were elaborate affairs with plenty of meat, including poultry, game, seafood, vegetable and fruit, followed up by a dessert. But the emphasis was on nonvegetarian dishes. This is the reason why lack of exercise started eroding the general health of people – who could afford to eat more, – in the 18th and 19th century. So, heart problems, as well as high blood pressure became quite common.

Grandmother knew how to tackle high blood pressure. She made sure that two bananas were fed without fail, to all her family members while they were in season. She did not know that the potassium content in the bananas counteracted the sodium content, brought about by a high salt intake.

If anybody suffered from high blood pressure and showed these symptoms – nosebleeds, severe anxiety and headaches and shortness of breath, – she knew that these symptoms were not conclusive, because she had never heard of the term high blood pressure.

Nevertheless, when any of her family members started displaying the symptoms, she immediately fed them bananas and honey. And if a person had a tendency to display the symptoms, she would immediately make up a mixture of five cloves of garlic, five leaves of the sacred basil and 4 teaspoons full of honey. She would then make the agitated and emotional patient eat this on an empty stomach, first thing in the morning.

Well, I guess she did not know that somebody would be suffering from a high blood pressure attack in the day, so she prevented this from happening by giving them this mixture, as soon as they got up. Also, the honey intake would make sure that the sugar levels in the blood were raised automatically, so the chances of a person suffering from high blood pressure was reduced drastically.

I do believe that grandma knew all about scientific procedures, and cause and effect without studying them. Besides, she knew that this knowledge had come down to her from her grandmother, and that is why children in the East are fed breakfasts with plenty of bananas, so that they do not suffer from blood pressure problems in the future.

Why Grandma Did Not Fuss

Grandmas have a tradition of being know all experienced, practical, lovable and caring women who are very popular with their grandchildren. In myth and fairytale, grandmas were the ones who fussed over and spoiled their grandchildren like Red Riding Hood and so on. In reality, grandmas were more practical. That was because they had hard days behind them, and they intended to pass on the knowledge to the generations coming after.

Curing Cuts, Bruises And Wounds

Grandma definitely did not believe in mollycoddling her children, because she was so busy controlling her household. That is why when a child came crying up to her, bleeding from a scraped knee or from a bloody and scratched face, which was the end result of childish scraps, she would not going to hysterics, and start yelling for a doctor for herself because she would not bear the sight of blood, especially when it was her own child hurt. [Believe me, I have seen a female do exactly that, and she terrified the child so much that it forgot that it was hurt and ran back to play, because its mother was screaming fit to beat the band. And he did not like noise.]

Grandma was more practical. She just washed the wound with potassium permanganate water, to get rid of the dirt and then sprinkled some powdered turmeric or powdered henna on the wound. After that, she gave the kiddie a swat on its posterior, and told it in a no-nonsense tone to go play, there was nothing wrong with it.

Nowadays, many of the parents I know do not have that sort of stoicism. They would rather call in a doctor, get tetanus shot injections, and fill the child up with antibiotics for every little scratch. I do not say that tetanus shot injections are not necessary – they prevent this dread disease from occurring, especially when the child has fallen among metal pieces or in an area well fertilized with organic manure especially horse manure. So if your child has cut itself really badly, go and see a doctor immediately. He is going to sew up the wound after disinfecting it properly.

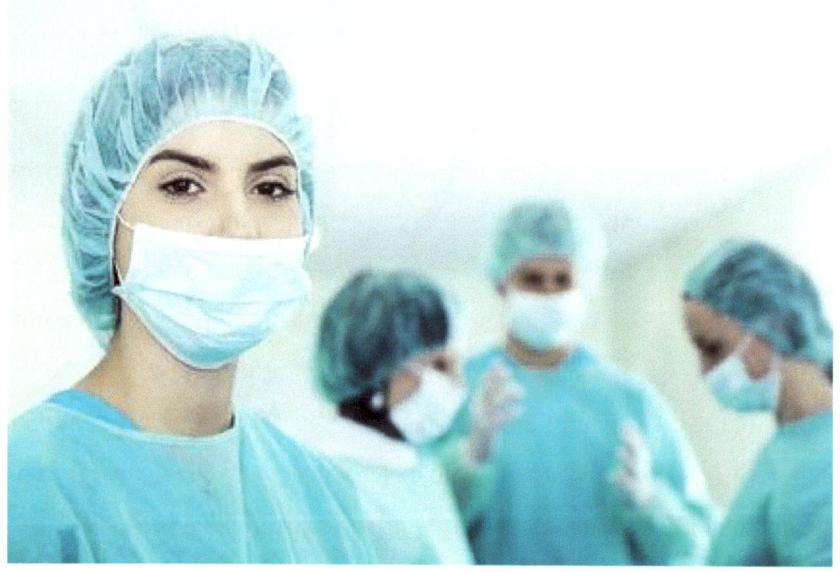

Remember, your doctor is your best friend, if you are badly hurt or injured.

Most of the time, children do not bother about getting their parents to clean their hearts, because according to them, parents fuss. Some parents get hysterical. Some parents say, "playing in such and such a place is definitely out of the question for you, young man", thus preventing the child from enjoying another source of enjoyable activity outdoors. In fact, the child is well on its way to get soft and mollycoddled, because mama is so protective.

Such a child is definitely not going to have a good auto immune system because it is going to be cooped up in ill ventilated rooms, close to mama. So if you happen to be that sort of fussy, finicky extra careful mama or Papa, are you making a pussycat out of your child? Do you prevent it from enjoying its childhood to the utmost, just because you are afraid that it might just scratch itself a bit or get a horrible tan or horrors, act like a child with other children?

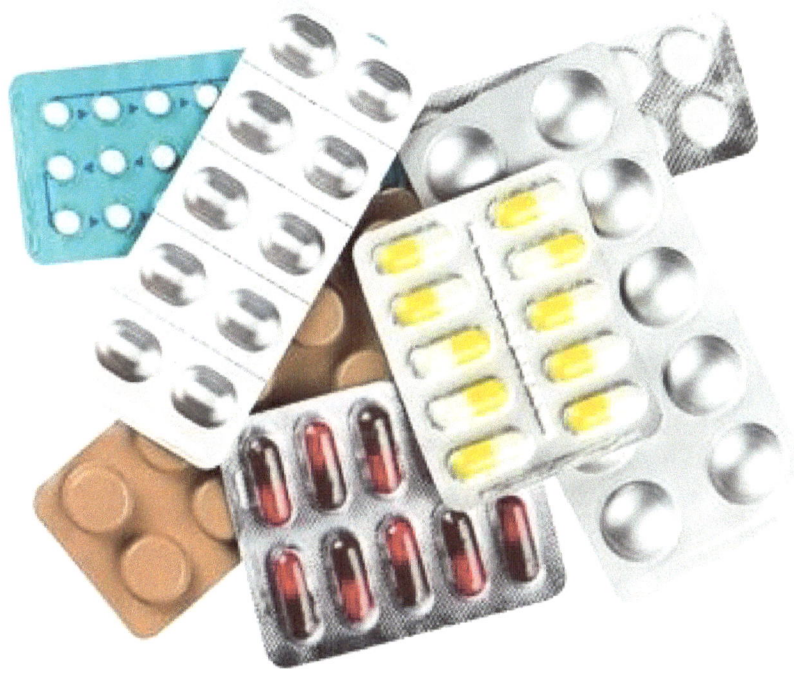

Remember that a healthy child is the child, which knows how to exercise its muscles by running, leaping, jumping, and exercising in the sun and fresh air during the age of growth – up to the age of nine. Otherwise, your child is going to be a fat, obese, sickly little porpoise with no physical staying power. And after that he is going to grow up into a tiresome adult, whining about his ill health, dosing himself with pills, because he has been brought upon them, and with absolutely no initiative to improve the state of ill health. Because after all, he is so used to mama and papa, taking care of him.

Do you know why so many of us cannot do without these pills? That is because we have been programmed since childhood to believe that they are the only things that can cure us and keep us healthy. Half the time, they are not necessary at all.

Grandma's children were self-reliant, and independent. They knew their disciplinary limits. They also knew how to enjoy life while they could, because when they grew up, they would have to work hard. But they knew all about the power of working hard since childhood, because grandma and grandpa never made their duties out to be a necessary burden which had to be done.

Instead, they taught by example. You would not see grandma lolling about in her kimono at 11 in the morning, because she had nothing useful or constructive to do. Instead, by 11, she would have done half a morning's work, getting up early to feed grandpa and the rest of the kids, who needed breakfast. After that, she took care of the house, went shopping, met her friends, worked in the garden, and on the whole, had a satisfactory constructive life and lifestyle.

Unfortunately, this is not so in the 21st century. Most of us really do not have the time to stop and stare. As for working in the garden, forget about it, we have a meeting to attend. We are very bothered about that promotion, and that is why we are going to work day and night to win in the rat race.

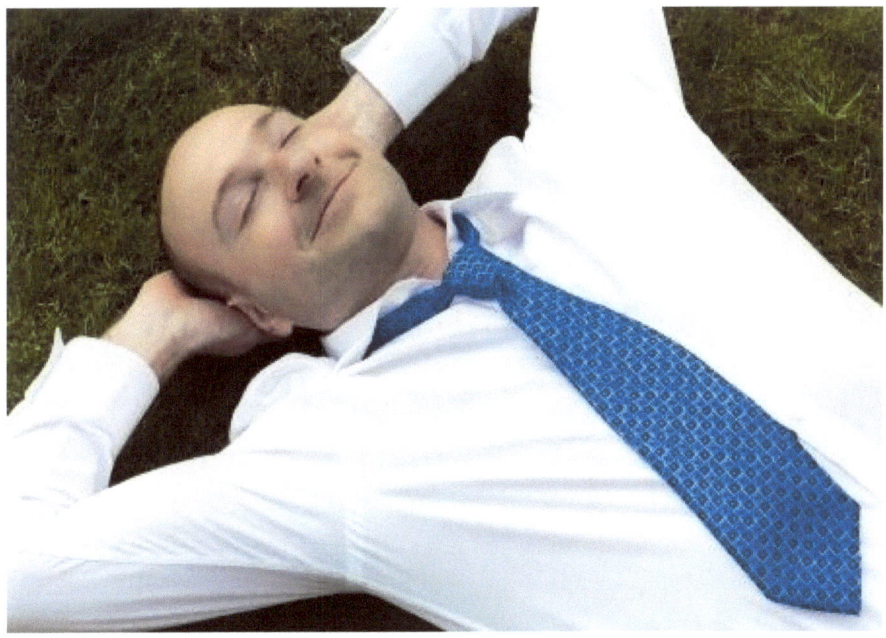

Is it any surprise that most of us come down with ill health, and ailments brought about through tension, stress and strain? So if you are suffering from depression, just because you feel low – try grandma's depression remedy.

Depression

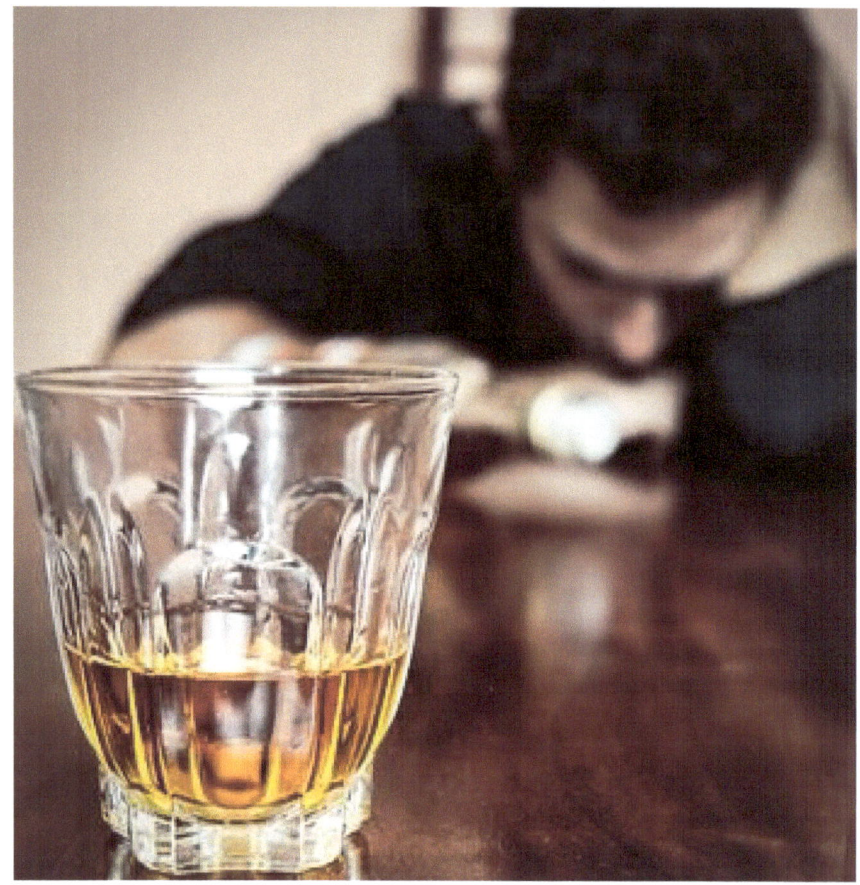

**People suffering from depression may become more dependent on
artificial stimulants like alcohol and depression management drugs.**

There is a remedy which has been used to cure depression since ancient
times. The ancient Egyptians had a surefire cure for depression. When
anybody began to think that life was not worth living, and he began to lose
interest in his surroundings, just because he had a surfeit of everything or

perhaps he was jealous because everybody else had a surfeit of everything, they had a really good cure for such a wet blanket.

He was immediately sent to the sea, under the care of a really nasty and strict sea captain. The sea captain would be annoying and crude enough to make his life "a thing of beauty and a joy,naah, never," by making him work physically from Dawn to dusk, in the open air. He would be fed bread with raw onions, salt and chilies. Amid this, he would be given a lecture about how soft he was, and how contemptible and burdensome and pestilential everybody found him, because he could not work with his hands in regular doses. He could not even help himself, because he was such a spineless jellyfish of a wimp.

Also, if the depression had reached the stage when a person became spiritless, the captain made sure that his family was insulted in his daily invigorating lectures. This in itself was enough for any proud person to retaliate. The moment he retaliated, he was considered to be cured of his depression, because he had regained his self-respect and interest in life. He was then brought back home, with the captain congratulating him about his new awakening, when he finally understood the meaning of his existence, his position in the scheme of things in society and in his family, and his responsibilities.

People of ancient civilizations believed depression to be one of the ways in which a person wanted to escape reality. Why do not the 21st century researchers think of this school of thought? Instead, we would rather sympathize with the person who is depressed, ask him to elaborate upon his ills – real and supposed – and so worsen his condition because he is now in complete "I need your pity" mode.

Grandma really did not have time to cajole a person out of what she called the sulks. Instead, she kept those people busy from morning to dusk, in hard physical labor, so that they did not have any chance or opportunity to sit in a corner and pity themselves.

Did you know that in medieval times, most of the people who suffered from depression were mostly of the upper classes? That was because they had time to sit, and brood over silly points, which were magnified in their minds out of all proportion.

Victor Hugo's daughter was one of them. She was an intelligent female, but she made herself into a case of depression through sheer "what do I do with myself, my father is the most well-known poet in France, and I really do not know how to continue in this boring existence. Ho-hum. What do I do today. I can languish languidly on this sofa, and not respond to anybody talking to me. Maybe then they will start talking about me." This was her way of trying to gain attention.

Many of the people suffering from depression may be just like Hugo's daughter. They are people bothered about themselves and according to them, the world should revolve around them. They quite enjoy the feeling of being pitied. On the other hand, there may be people really suffering from genetic depression and these people need immediate psychological care.

Do not take depression lightly. At the same time, do not make the patient feel that he is going to spend the rest of his life being supported by you, because you positively revel in the feeling that you are taking care of a person who is depressed, and you are the only one who can manage him.

Believe it or not, as a psychologist I found just this case in my neighborhood. The person got depressed because his mother positively enjoyed the sensation of telling everybody that she was taking care of her depressed child and she was such a good mom, and only she could understand his sensitive nature.

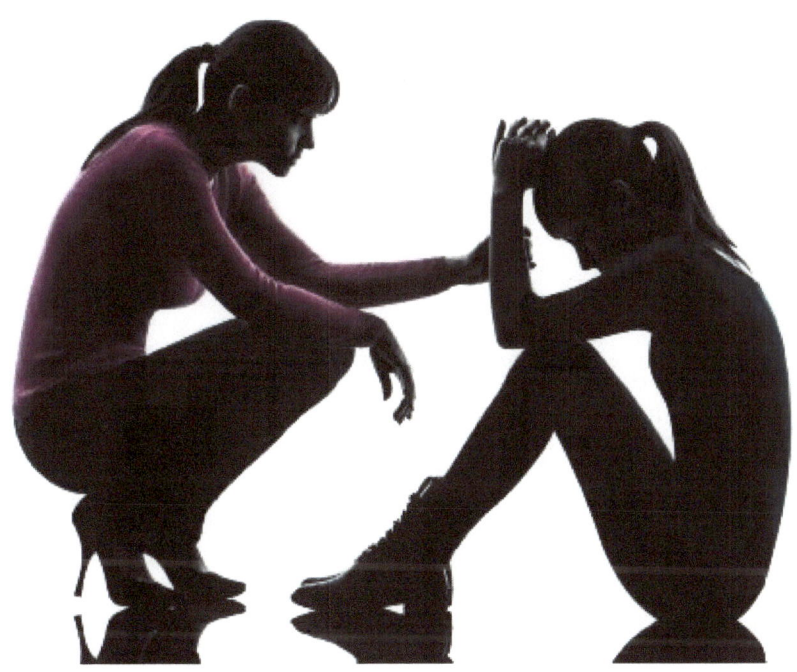

There may be some genuine reason behind this apathy. There may also be a cry for help, a bid for attention, or perhaps some other reason for this state in human beings.

That silly woman ruined a perfectly good and healthy psyche, just because she wanted some excitement in her life. The boy was a very intelligent and well balanced extrovert. Also, being a normal, healthy young human boy he was subject to normal growing up pains, and sulks, when he would not want to communicate with his very inquisitive and curious mom. These according to the mother were signs of depression, because she heard from someone that those were surefire depression symptoms. The poor imaginative boy began to think that he was really suffering from depression.

Can you imagine the horror of such a mental state, brought about by the foolishness of one not so intelligent brain playing on a much more intelligent brains psyche, psychology, and emotional well-being?

If anybody in grandma's circle suffered from depression, she would immediately attribute it to some imbalance in the body and mind. She would then cure it by boiling ¼ teaspoon of green cardomom seeds in light tea water and feed it to the patient. She would also makes 1/8 teaspoon of powdered nutmeg with the one tablespoon of fresh gooseberry juice. This would be given to the depressed person three times a day. This also is a good remedy for people suffering from **irritability**.

Along with that, she would accompany this dosing with "that is enough of mooching around, get off your lazy posterior, and give us a hand, you are not the Queen of Sheba" and other such rough words. Grandma was a caution she was, and would not stop at just words, but would also give such a "moocher," [in her light] a heavy tap on the Dignity area, to get the person moving.

We would not do that. We are so extremely civilized. We would rather send our children to psychologists, because it is the stylish thing to do. We would also not bother about disciplining them, because they need to find their own individuality and express it in every way they can. And then we come down with nervous breakdowns, because our children are spoiled intolerable brats.

Nervous Problems

So if you are suffering from nervous problems, resulting from stress and strain, drink an infusion of 2 tablespoons chopped mint leaves steeped in one cup of water for 30 minutes and drink it down with one teaspoonful of honey.This helps tone your system, especially when you find yourself being stressed.

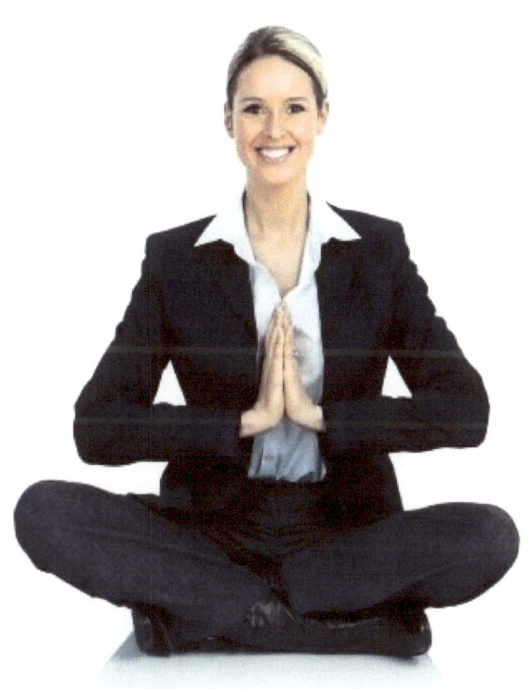

Meditation can be a great stress buster

Obesity Cure

I am giving you some remedies for obesity, but if you persist on no exercise and plenty of junk food, well, that is your outlook.

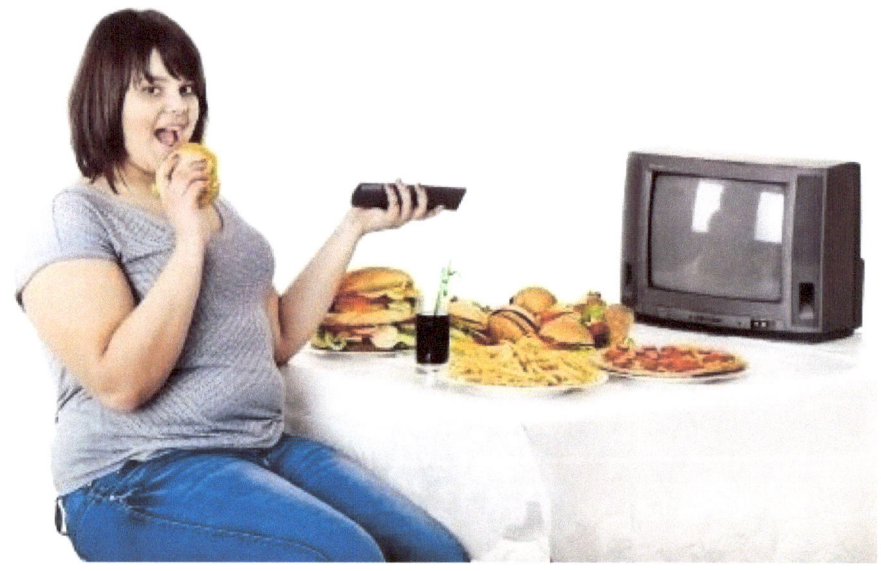

Eating junk food does not help to control or manage obesity.

Nevertheless, if you intend to change your lifestyle, watch your diet, and you are sure that you are not suffering from genetic obesity, you can manage to control it naturally. This was done in ancient times, when obese people were given 1 teaspoon lime juice in a cup of water, followed by one tomato first thing in the morning on an empty stomach.

Curry leaves

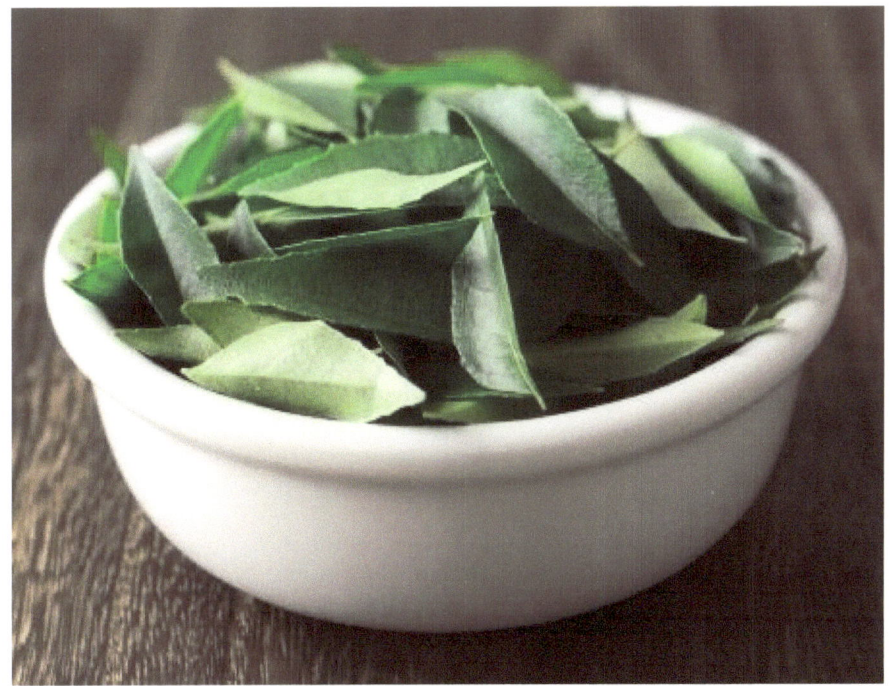

In India, especially in the South of India, I saw one of my naturopath friends, eating 10 fresh fully grown curry leaves every morning for 3 to 4 months. He said that that controlled obesity. But then, curry leaves are an important part of South Indian cuisine, put in every dish. Is that the reason why they are so fit and trim? Believe me, diet has everything to do with it.

Lemon Juice Regime

Also, you may try out this three months obesity control regime. Mix 1 teaspoon of three teaspoons lemon juice, with four powdered peppercorns with 1 teaspoon honey in a cup of water. Drink this first thing in the morning for three months. I have known people losing weight with these methods – you can use any of them – but I would suggest also supplementing this natural cure with some form of physical exercise.

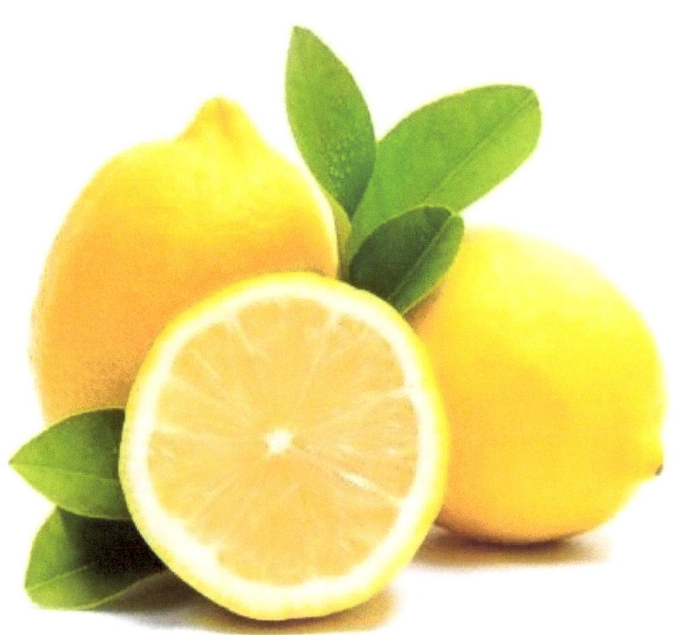

Losing weight Through Exercise? How Boring!

Do you know why our ancestors were so healthy? That is because they worked hard throughout the day. They never had time to sit down and relax. They definitely did not have time to sit in one place, continuously for eight hours in a day, scrunched up like a sponge and thus gaining weight in the waist and upper leg regions.

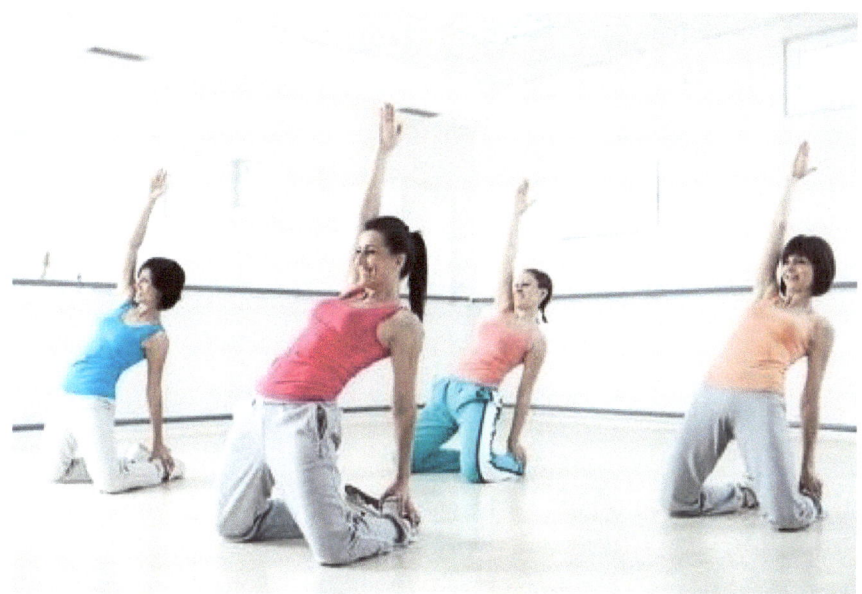

This physical activity was not called exercise. It was called work. However, as lifestyles changed in the 20th and 21st century, physical labor became an obsolete necessary for a majority of us. We were called upon to do work which needed mental exercise. That is why we began to resort to exercise routines and workouts to keep ourselves fit. Is not this an irony? What came naturally to our ancestors, during a normal day's work was being repeated by their descendants through artificial and expensive methods in stuffy rooms under artificial light.

Many of us began to hate the word of exercise, because according to us, that meant getting sweaty, and tired. That was because we had forgotten how to pace ourselves. We exhausted our bodies on the very day of the very first day of our routine, trying to prove to ourselves that we were still as fit now as we were in our 20s. The aching muscles at night, and the next morning proved that it was not so. Naturally, the signal went to the brain, that exercise was extremely painful. So we began to shirk it.

I belong to this category. I would rather sit than walk about, take the lift instead of climbing up the stairs, because tiring my muscles is so boring. So if you belong to this category here are some tips, with which you can keep fit and also lose some weight. Hopefully, your mind is going to be ready for an exercise routine, which is pleasurable and is definitely not a duty.

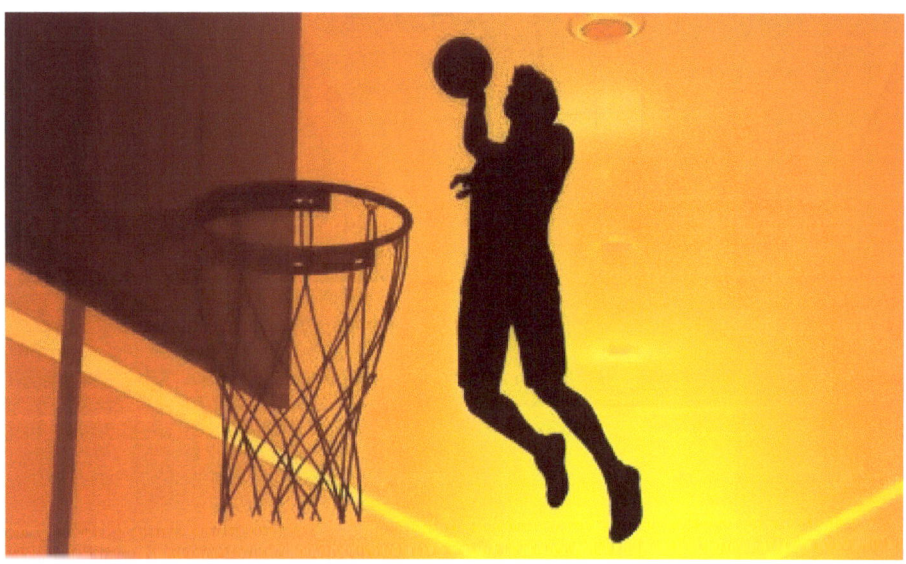

Get your metabolism working. Once it gets used to the idea that you are going to subject the body to some sort of exercise, it is going to be prepared for that exercise. Never do any sort of exercise, which strains your body. Let me tell you this sad sad story. After the necessary regime of compulsory games at college, I promised myself that I would never, ever exercise for "the pride of the college", as long as I lived, unless I enjoyed doing that activity. Playing physical games as a duty or because you are a responsible member of a team, and have to play the game, is the most painful activity of student life. So that meant that within 10 years, my athletic physique had gone back to flabby, with bad muscle tone. Though I never gained fat, I was badly out of condition.

Then one day, when I was channel surfing, I saw a dance program, where people were being taught how to dance. I noticed that every step which was being done was a part of an exercise regime, which I knew from school and college days. But the ponytailed instructor was doing those dance steps to the sound of music. And everybody was enjoying that work out.
Now I understood the meaning of autosuggestion. If I had been told to exercise to lose weight and get fit, yawn, what a bore. On the other hand, if my weight loss instructor had told us that he/she was not a weight-loss instructor, but a dance instructor, who would get us fit and fine in three months, see how many people would have enrolled in his/her classes – me included –.

It is all a matter of looking at things. So if you have a problem in keeping fit, just because you do not want to exercise, look for some activity which gets you out in the fresh air, at least once a day . I enjoy walking, swimming, and ha ha, "dancing", because my muscles are getting a chance to stretch and grow and develop. You may want to try out something, which you like.
Do not reject an idea out of hand before you have tried it. Believe me, I really could not dance, till I reached my 40s. And then, my mind acknowledged the fact that every dance gesture was a part of an exercise routine or a yoga routine. You just needed to synchronize it according to

what your body wanted you to do, when the music was on. In two weeks, I learned how to dance on my own, because the body was working in synchronization with the mind, which ordered the different parts to do one particular action, while another part of the body did another action. Then repeat thrice and then try something else, with the involvement of more parts of your body.

Believe me, this is hilarious, enjoyable, and really good fun. Also, it meant that I lost weight without even knowing it. 15 minutes a day. Not more. You may find yourself extending these enjoyable sessions from 15 to 30. Do not be like Gene Kelly, practicing eight hours continuously, because he was such a perfectionist. Do not exercise for more than 30 minutes in one session.

Conclusion

So here you are with volume 4 of grandma's ancient remedies and herbal recipes, with tips, rules of living, good advice, and also natural cures. People in the 21st century are getting to know more and more about natural therapy as alternative medicine, because that is proved effective.

In the same manner, they are looking for ways and means in which they can change their lifestyles. Sedentary living is slowly going out of fashion. More people are trying to incorporate some sort of physical exercise, during the day in order to keep fit and healthy. So you may want to look at all the tips and techniques, given in this fourth volume.

Along with that, you are going to find the knowledge of the ancients, which was used to heal people in all walks of life. Fruit, vegetables and spices along with minerals, were used to make up these remedies. Most of these remedies, especially those written in a Egyptian papyri and more than 3000 years old definitely do not stand up to the light of scientific reasoning and Advanced Technology. Incantations and chants do not cure diseases or heal you. Nor do exotic witches brews made up of crocodile skin and a marigold flower gathered under the light of the full moon after it has been cut with a silver knife, going to help heal common ailments.

The Egyptian, Persian and Babylonian priests were considered to be very knowledgeable. They also had to keep the hoi polloi under control. So they knew the necessary ingredients, which would help cure an ailment. They would garb and disguise that particular ingredient in a covering of superficial items like flowers, fruits, and herbs. And as they were showmen, they would ask the patient to do some chants.

So when that patient was cured, he would go around praising the priests as well as the Gods to whom he had asked the priests to sacrifice three white hens or a goat along with the offering of one gold ring to those kind Immortals. [What did the priests eat, well cooked and seasoned in exotic spices that day? So asks this cynic.]

Many of the natural herbal remedies and recipes, which have thus come down the ages are quack remedies. However, among them, there are some remedies, which are really effective, and do cure the patient. It is going to take a knowledgeable person to interpret these remedies. This was how the priests kept their knowledge to themselves.

The people in their own medical circles knew the gold from the dross. So even if the papyri got into the hands of the ignorant, they would be very well pleased, with all the extra incantations and rare ingredients, which went into the making of potions, because that convinced them how knowledgeable their priests really were.

Nevertheless, the remedies given here are totally time-tested, and have been used. They are not quack remedies. So if you believe in the healing power of fruit, vegetables, spices and natural remedies, this is the book for you. Keep healthy the natural way!

Author Bio

Dueep Jyot Singh is a Management and IT Professional who managed to gather Postgraduate qualifications in Management and English and Degrees in Science, French and Education while pursuing different enjoyable career options like being an hospital administrator, IT,SEO and HRD Database Manager/ soft skills trainer, movie and radio scriptwriter, theatre artiste and public speaker, lecturer in French, Marketing and Advertising, ex-Editor of Hearts On Fire (now known as Solsctice) Books Missouri USA, advice columnist and cartoonist, publisher and Aviation School trainer, ex-moderator on Medico.in, banker, student councilor,travelogue writer … among other things! One fine morning, she decided that she had enough of killing herself by Degrees and went back to her first love -- writing. It's more enjoyable! She already has 48 published academic and 14 fiction- in- different- genre books under her belt.

When she is not designing websites or making Graphic design illustrations for clients she is busy browsing in old bookshops for antique books,-she has a mouthwatering collection of priceless First editions and rare books…including R.L. Stevenson, O.Henry, Dornford Yates, Maurice Walsh, C.N.Williamson, and the crown of her collection- Dickens "The Old Curiosity Shop," and so on… Just call her "Renaissance Woman" - collecting herbal remedies, making one of a kind creations in Irish Crochet and Aran knitting, acting like Universal Helping Hand/Agony Aunt, or escaping to her dear forests and mountains for a bit of exploring, collecting herbs and plants and trekking.

Check out some of the other JD-Biz Publishing books

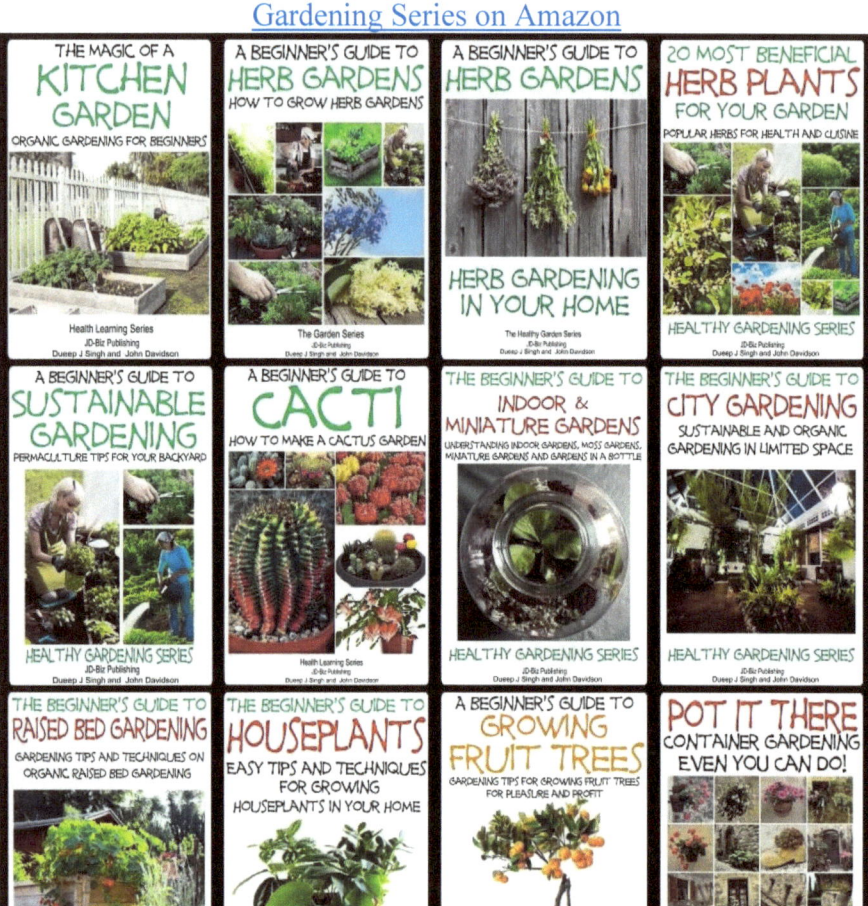

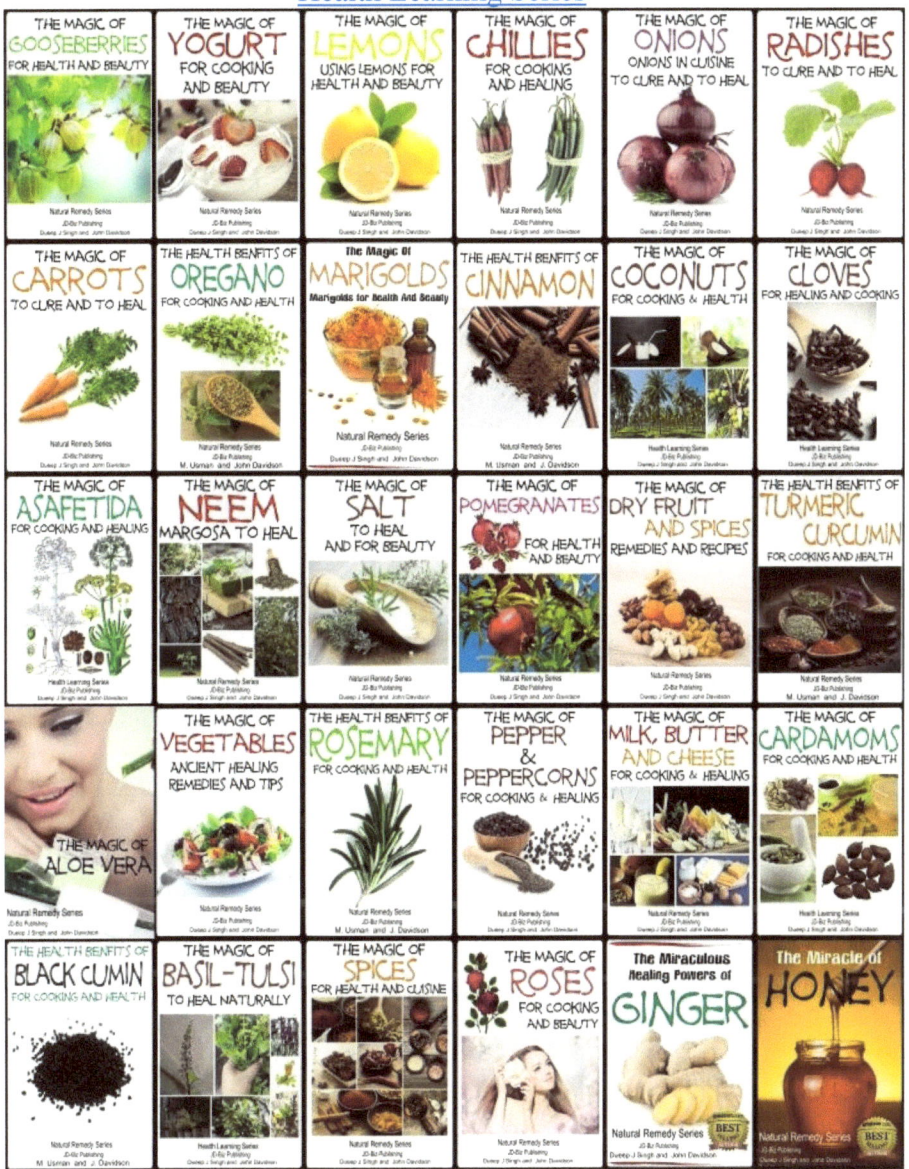

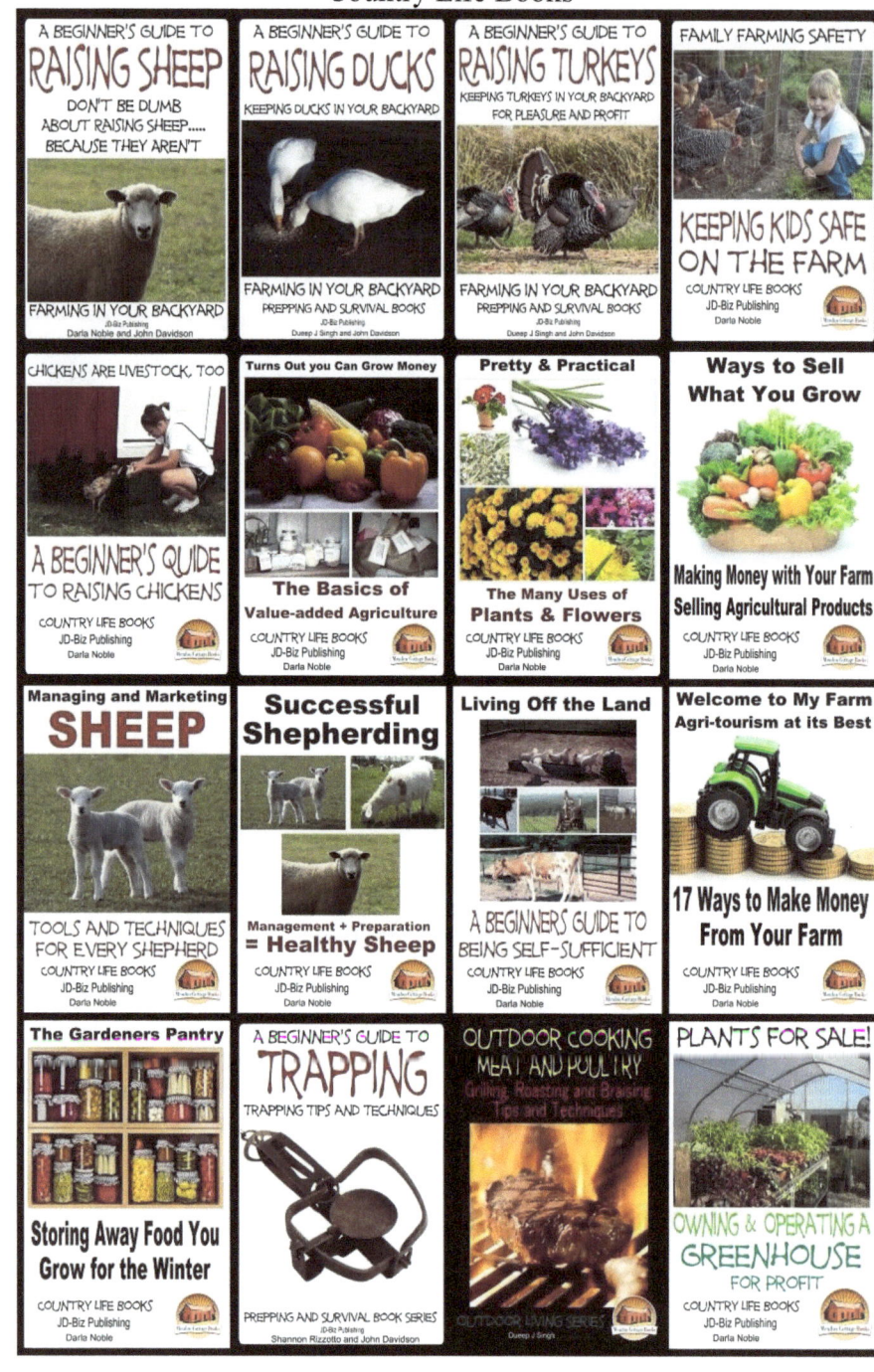

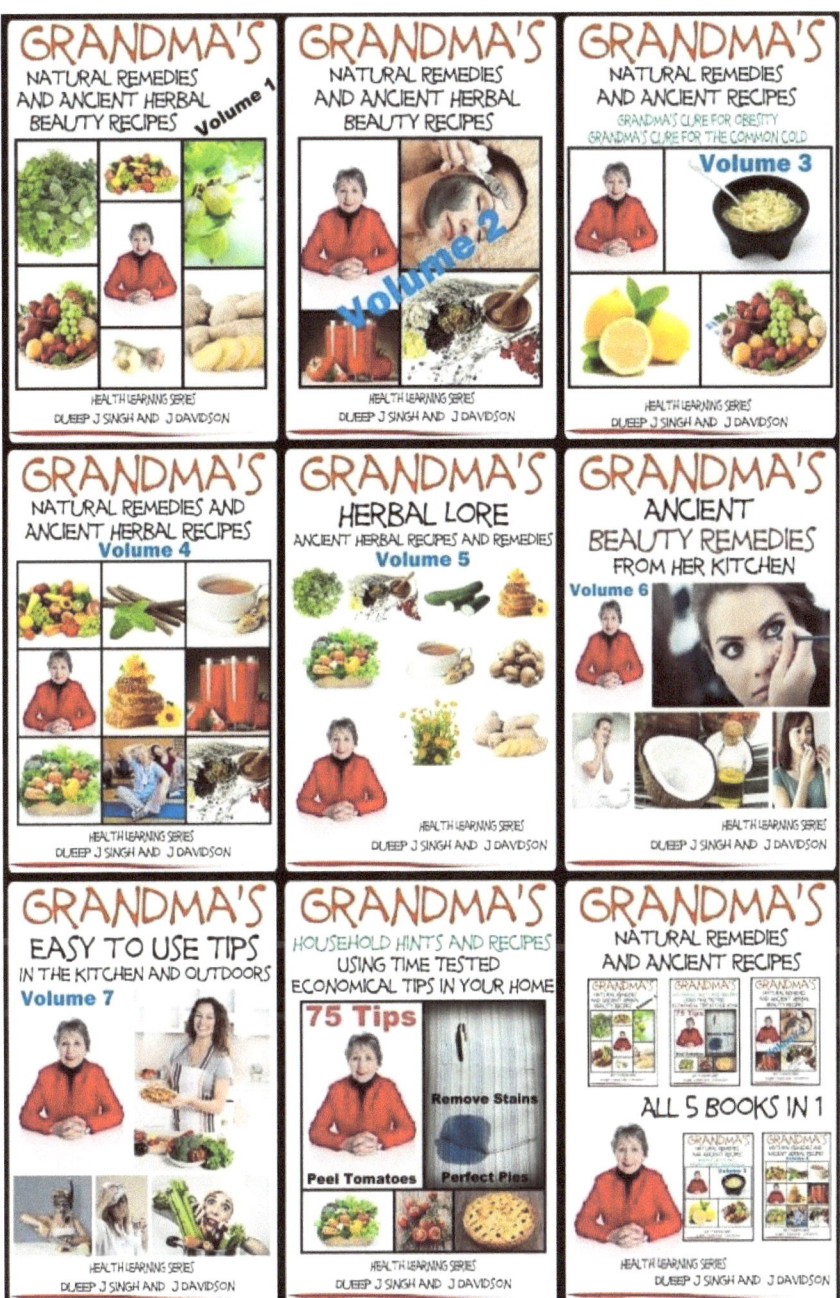

Health Learning Series

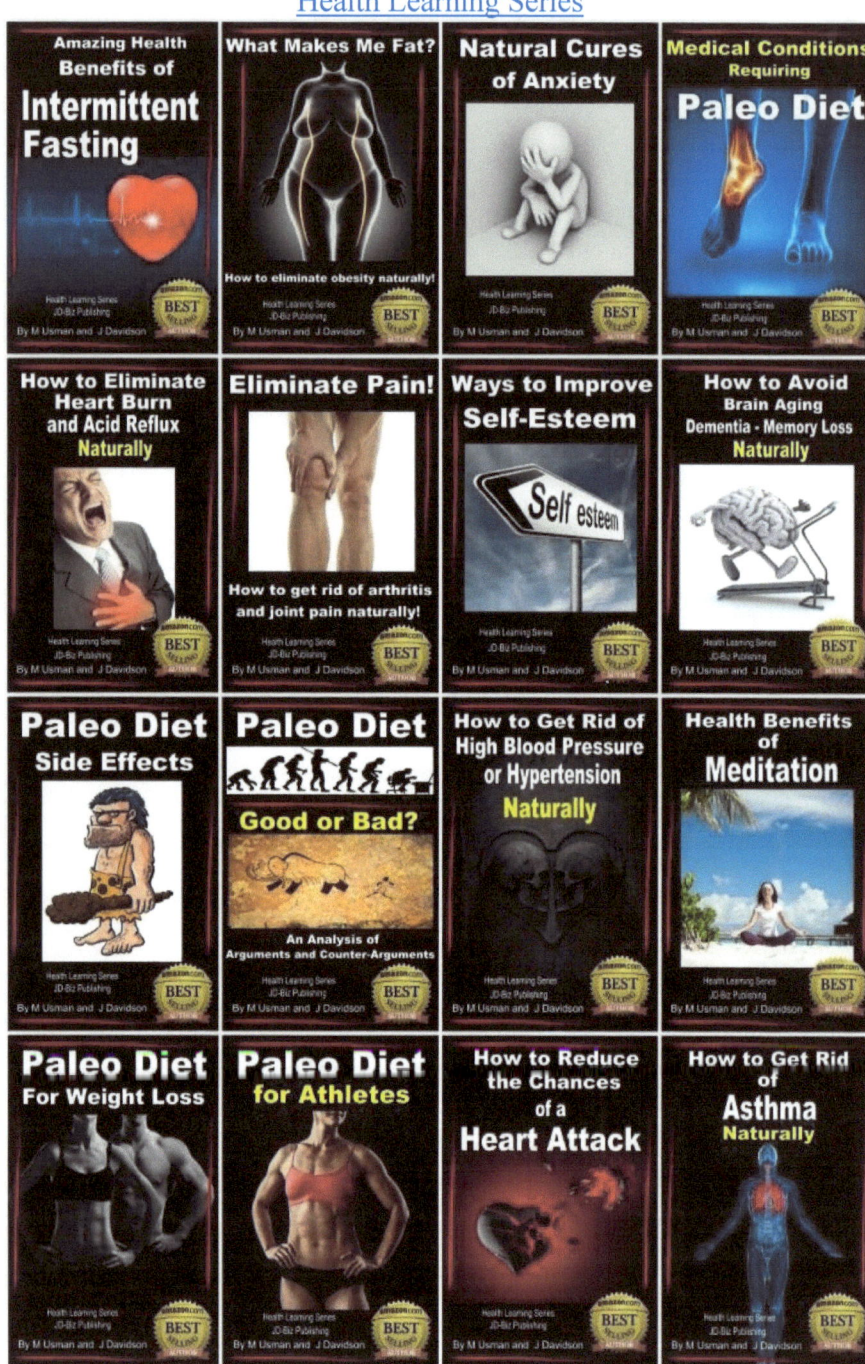

Amazing Animal Book Series

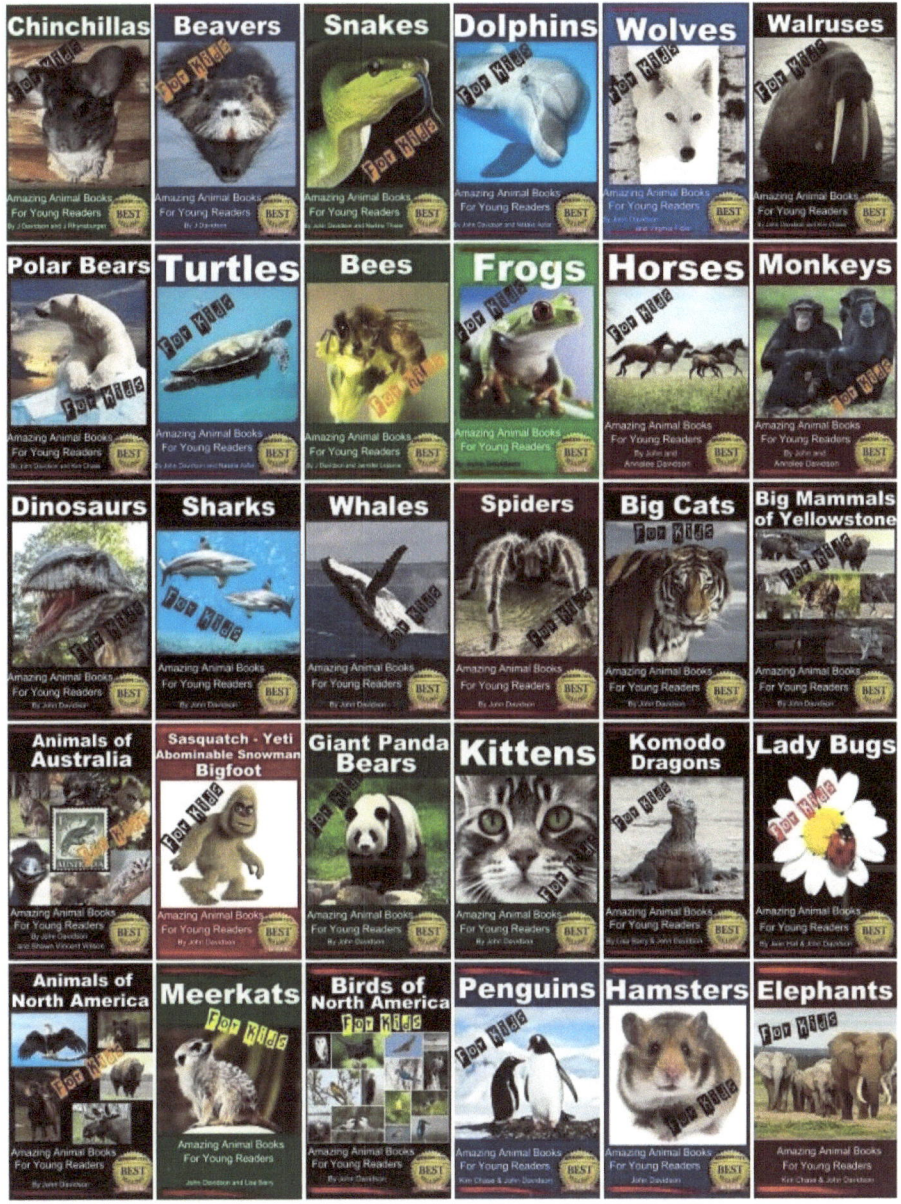

Learn To Draw Series

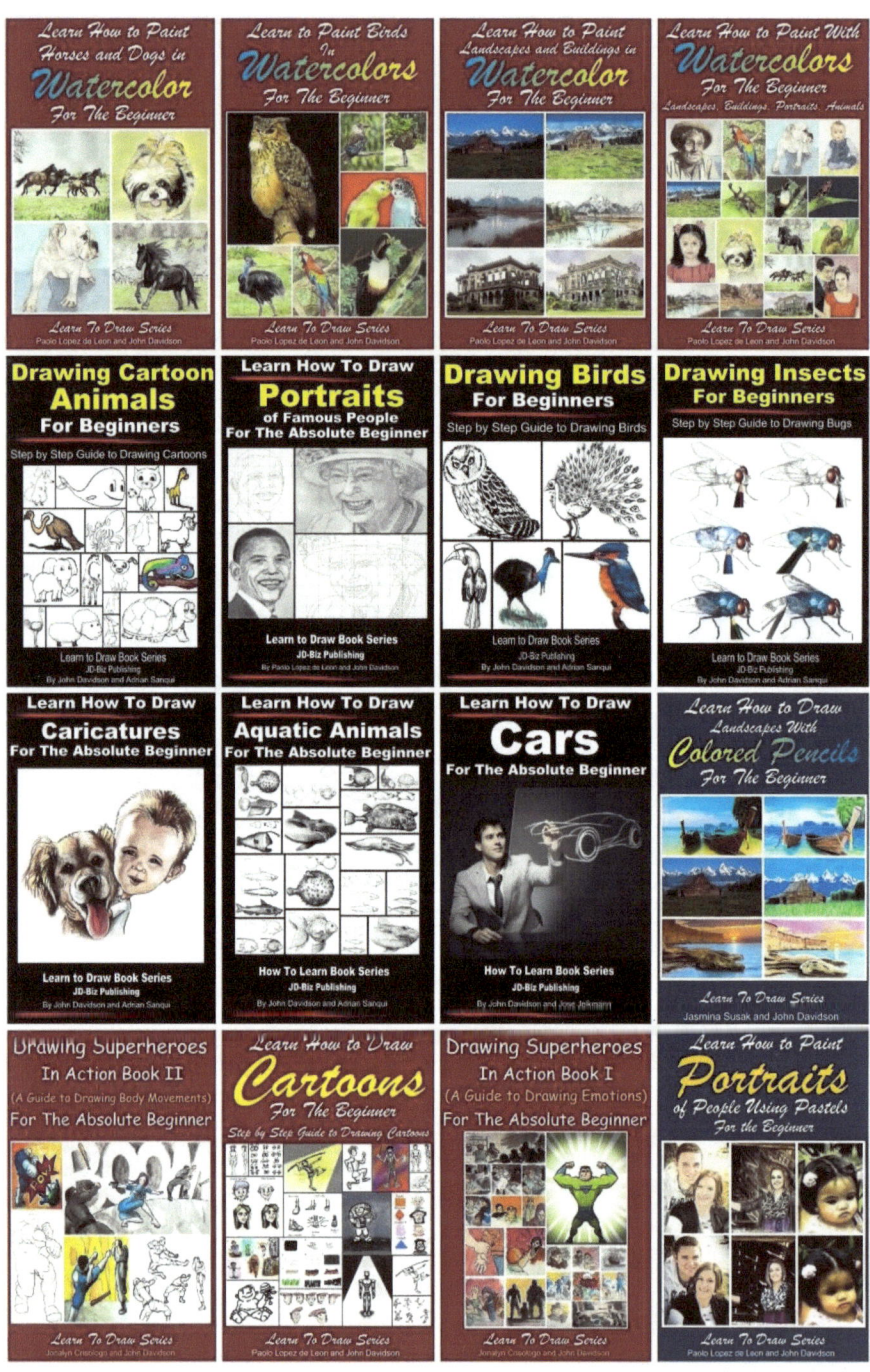

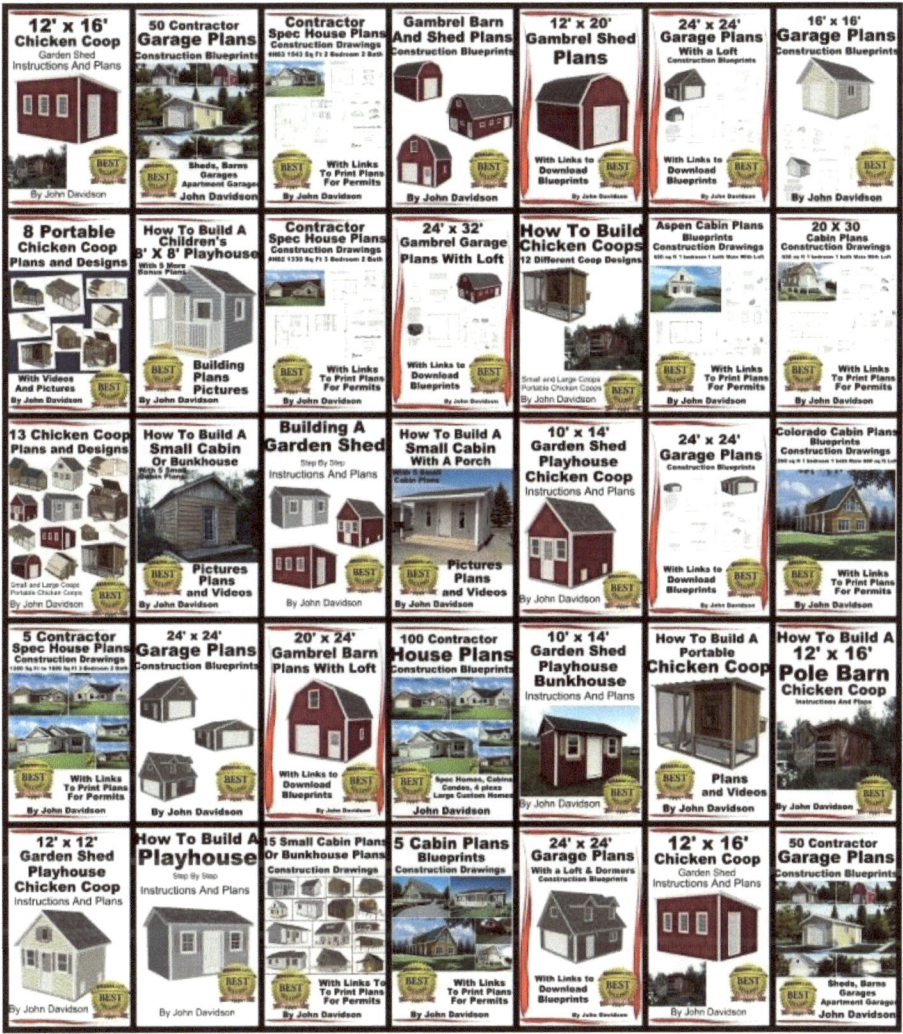

Entrepreneur Book Series

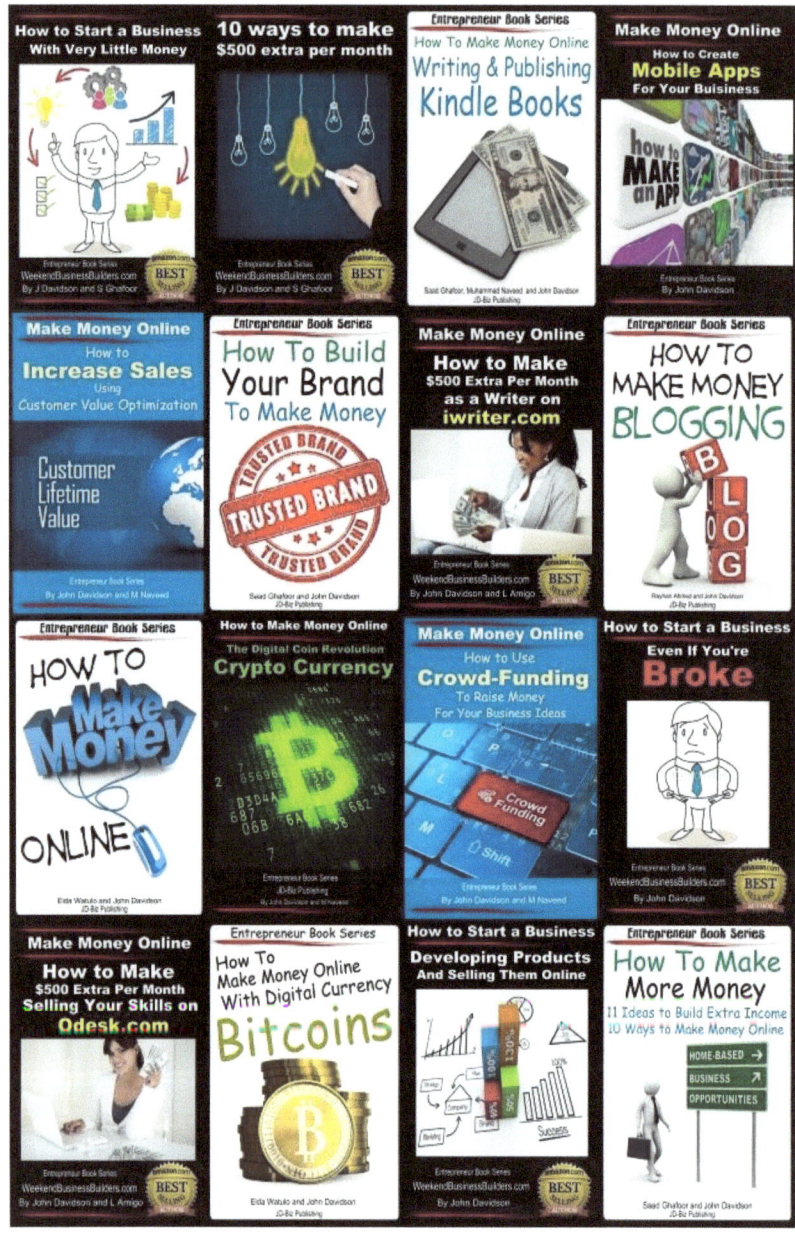

Our books are available at

1. Amazon.com

2. Barnes and Noble

3. Itunes

4. Kobo

5. Smashwords

6. Google Play Books

Download Free Books!

http://MendonCottageBooks.com

Publisher

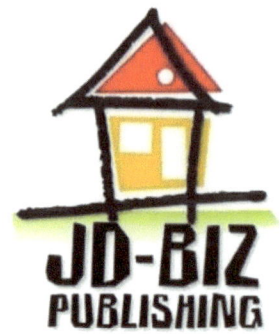

JD-Biz Corp

P O Box 374

Mendon, Utah 84325

http://www.jd-biz.com/

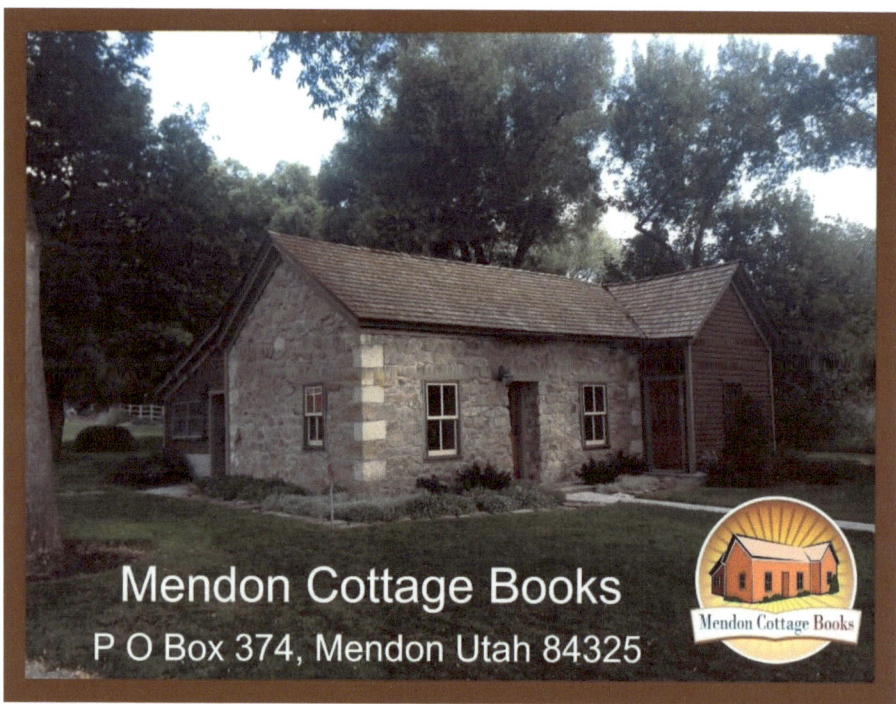

Mendon Cottage Books

P O Box 374, Mendon Utah 84325

www.ingramcontent.com/pod-product-compliance
Lightning Source LLC
Chambersburg PA
CBHW050822290526
45792CB00001B/221